FREEDOM FROM DEPRESSION FOREVER!

A THERAPY THAT WORKS FOR MEN

BY
IHEKE WILLIAMS

COPYRIGHT © 2019, IHEKE WILLIAMS

All rights reserved under International Copyright Law. Contents and/or cover may not be reproduced in whole or in part in any form without the express written permission of Iheke Williams.

Unless otherwise indicated, all scripture quotations are taken from the King James Version of the Bible A key for other Bible versions used

NKJV	New King James Version
AMP	The Amplified Bible
TANT	The New Amplified Bible
TLB -	The Living Bible
CEV -	Contemporary English Version
NASB	New American Standard Version
GW -	God's Word version
ESV -	English Standard Version
NET -	New English Translation
ISV -	International Standard Version
NIV -	New International Version
MSG -	The Message Translation

DEDICATION

This Book is dedicated to Almighty God and to everyone in the world.

TABLE OF CONTENT

DIVINE HEALTH AFFIRMATIONS AGAINST DEPRESSION
COPYRIGHT © 2019, IHEKE WILLIAMS
DEDICATION
TABLE OF CONTENT
WHAT IS DEPRESSION?
WHAT IS GOD'S SOLUTION
INSTRUCTION 1
INSTRUCTION 2
DAY 1
DAY 2
DAY 3
DAY 4
DAY 5
DAY 6
DAY 7
DAY 8
DAY 9
DAY 10
DAY 11
DAY 12
DAY 13
DAY 14
DAY 15
DAY 16
DAY 17
DAY 18
DAY 19
DAY 20
DAY 21
DAY 22
DAY 23
DAY 24
DAY 25
DAY 26
DAY 27
DAY 28
DAY 29
DAY 30
DAY 31
SUMMARY
PRAYER FOR SALVATION
OTHER INFORMATION
ABOUT THE AUTHOR

WHAT IS DEPRESSION?

Major depressive disorder(MDD), also known simply as **depression**, is a mental disorder characterized by at least two weeks of low mood that is present across most situations.

It is often accompanied by low self-esteem, loss of interest in normally enjoyable activities, low energy, and pain without a clear cause. People may also occasionally have false beliefs or see or hear things that others cannot

Source: Wikipedia

WHAT IS GOD'S SOLUTION

"...By His wounds ye have been healed.." – 1 Peter 2:24

JESUS has already healed you over 2000 years ago on the cross.

You have NO business with depression. Don't allow Satan to deceive you that your life is worthless and that you have nothing to live for. Satan will bring events and pictures to your mind to try to convince you that you are useless, worthless and should die. Those images are not from God, Don't listen to Satan or his demons. Don't listen to demons. They are liars. Demons hate us all, they want to "...steal, kill and destroy.." - – John 10:10. Jesus has saved us Already – 1 Peter 2:24.

Your life was healed over 2000 years ago on the cross. Your life is in Christ now and it is Active, Fruitful, Productive and Strong, right now. No devil can take that away from you. Don't allow demons to ruin your life.

You will affirm this blessing in your life for 31 days and FOREVER!

INSTRUCTION 1

That if thou shalt confess with thy mouth the Lord Jesus, and shalt believe in thine heart that God hath raised him from the dead, thou shalt be saved. – Romans 10:9

There has to be a connection with what you say and what you have in your heart. We believe with our heart, this is the reason you have to meditate on the gospel with your heart, believe it and then affirm it with your mouth.

For the affirmations to be effective, you will have to meditate on the scripture (1Peter 2:24) for 5 minutes, in your heart, and then affirm it with your mouth.

INSTRUCTION 2

"For our light affliction, which is but for a moment, worketh for us a far more exceeding and eternal weight of glory;

<u>While we look not at the things which are seen</u>, but at the things which are not seen: for the things which are seen are temporal; but the things which are not seen are eternal. –
2 Corinthians 4:17-18

Don't look at the mirror or yourself during the duration of the affirmation. It affects the word in your heart when you keep seeing the effects of the depression on your body.

Do not touch any part of your body that has been affected by this depression.

Don't talk about depression. Only affirm the Blessings you received from the Lord Jesus Christ on the cross in 1 Peter 2:24

Follow these instructions and your affirmations will be more effective.

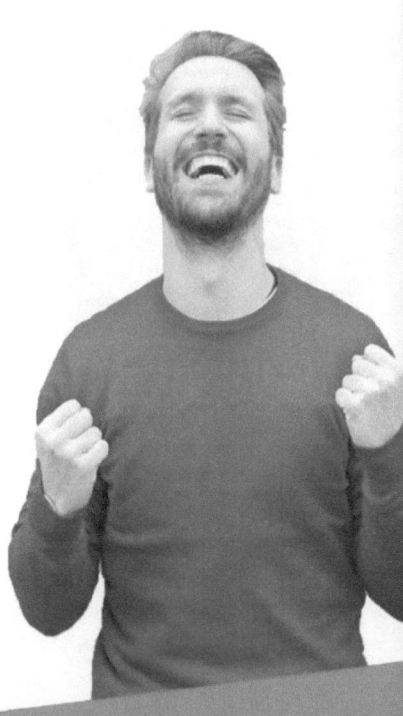

DAY 1
AFFIRMATION

Meditate on 1 Peter 2:24B in your heart for 5 minutes

"..By His stripes ye have been healed.."

Now say the words below to yourself

"I HAVE BEEN HEALED THEREFORE, I AFFIRM THAT I AM NOT DEPRESSED!"

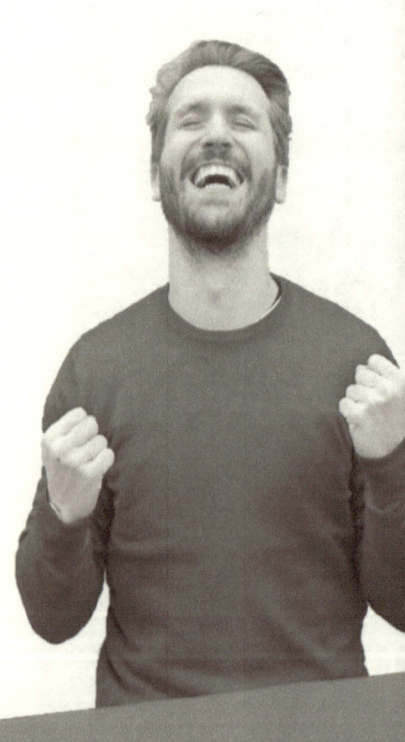

DAY 2
AFFIRMATION

Meditate on 1 Peter 2:24B in your heart for 5 minutes

"..By His stripes ye have been healed.."

Now say the words below to yourself

"I HAVE BEEN HEALED THEREFORE, I AFFIRM THAT I AM ACTIVE AND STRONG FOREVER!"

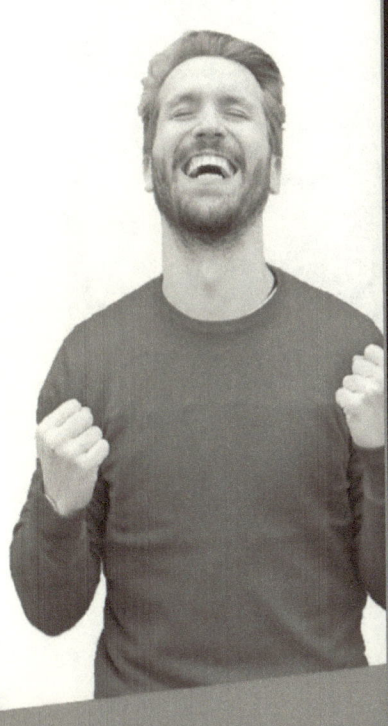

DAY 3
AFFIRMATION

Meditate on 1 Peter 2:24B in your heart for 5 minutes

"..By His stripes ye have been healed.."

Now say the following words to yourself

"I HAVE BEEN HEALED THEREFORE, I AFFIRM THAT MY FUTURE IS ACTIVE AND BLESSED FOREVER!"

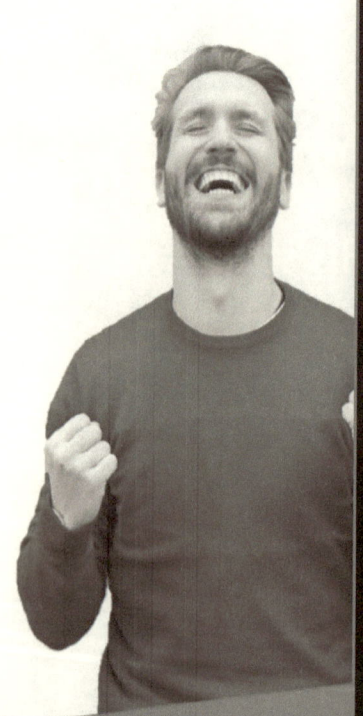

DAY 4 AFFIRMATION

Meditate on 1 Peter 2:24B in your heart for 5 minutes

"..By His stripes ye have been healed.."

Now say the words below to yourself

"I HAVE BEEN HEALED THEREFORE, I AFFIRM THAT MY MIND IS FREE FROM ALL DEMONIC INFLUENCES FOREVER!"

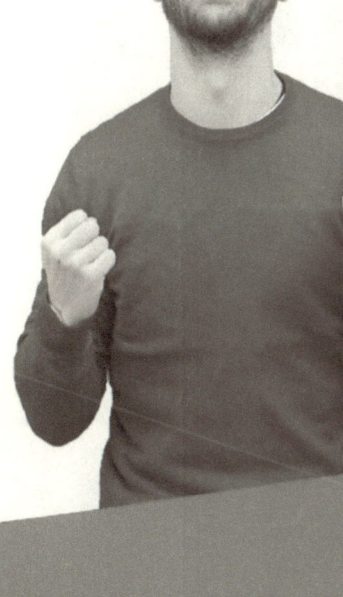

DAY 5 AFFIRMATION

Meditate on 1 Peter 2:24B in your heart for 5 minutes

"..By His stripes ye have been healed.."

Now say the words below to yourself

"MY FAMILY HAVE BEEN HEALED THEREFORE, I AFFIRM THAT MY FAMILY IS BLESSED, ACTIVE AND STRONG FOREVER!"

DAY 6
AFFIRMATION

Meditate on 1 Peter 2:24B in your heart for 5 minutes

"..By His stripes ye have been healed.."

Now say the words below to yourself

"I HAVE BEEN HEALED THEREFORE, I AFFIRM THAT I AM ACTIVE AND STRONG FOREVER!"

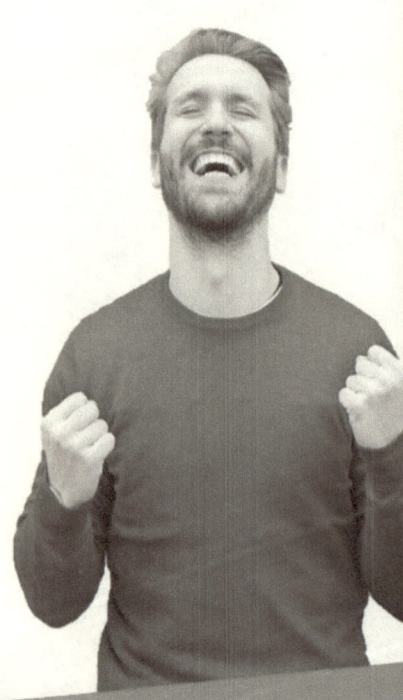

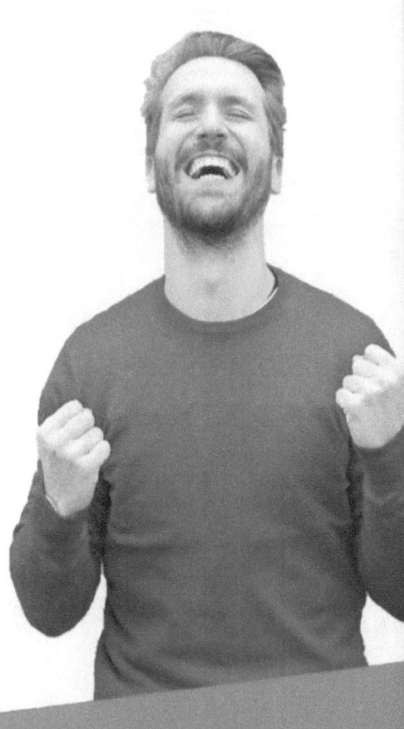

DAY 7
AFFIRMATION

Meditate on 1 Peter 2:24B in your heart for 5 minutes

"..By His stripes ye have been healed.."

Now say the words below to yourself

"I HAVE BEEN HEALED THEREFORE, I AFFIRM THAT I AM NOT DEPRESSED!"

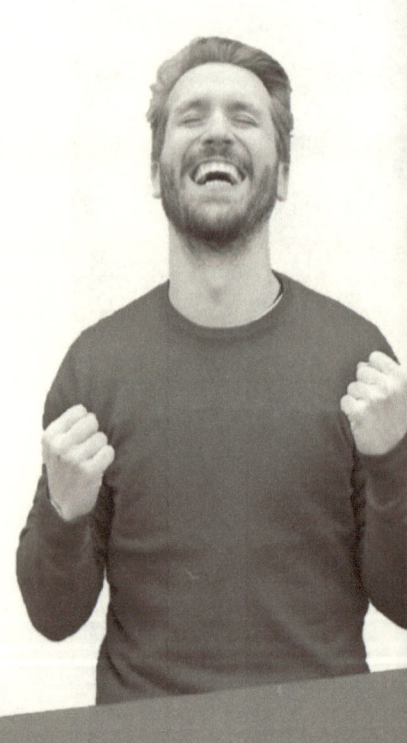

DAY 8
AFFIRMATION

Meditate on 1 Peter 2:24B in your heart for 5 minutes

"..By His stripes ye have been healed.."

Now say the words below to yourself

"I HAVE BEEN HEALED THEREFORE, I AFFIRM THAT MY LIFE IS ACTIVE AND BLESSED FOREVER!"

DAY 9
AFFIRMATION

Meditate on 1 Peter 2:24B in your heart for 5 minutes

"..By His stripes ye have been healed.."

Now say the words below to yourself

"I HAVE BEEN HEALED THEREFORE, I AFFIRM THAT MY FUTURE IS ACTIVE AND BLESSED FOREVER!"

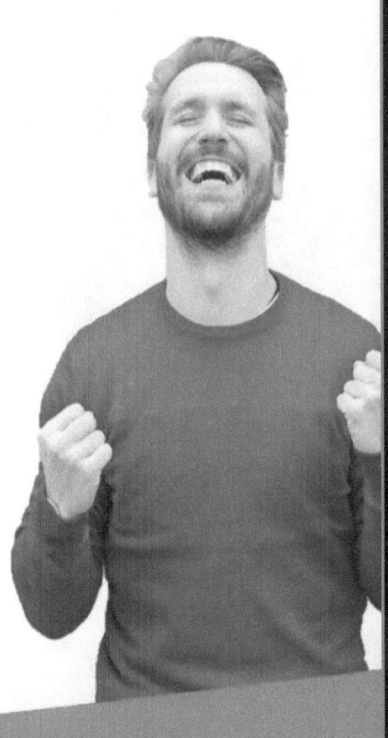

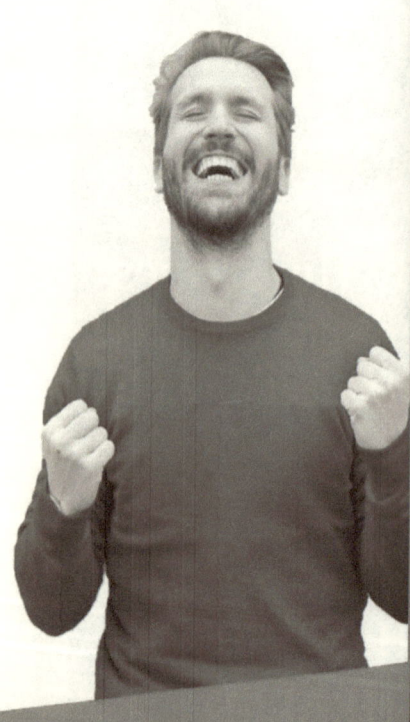

DAY 10
AFFIRMATION

Meditate on 1 Peter 2:24B in your heart for 5 minutes

"..By His stripes ye have been healed.."

Now say the words below to yourself

"I HAVE BEEN HEALED THEREFORE, I AFFIRM THAT SATAN CANNOT DESTROY ME!"

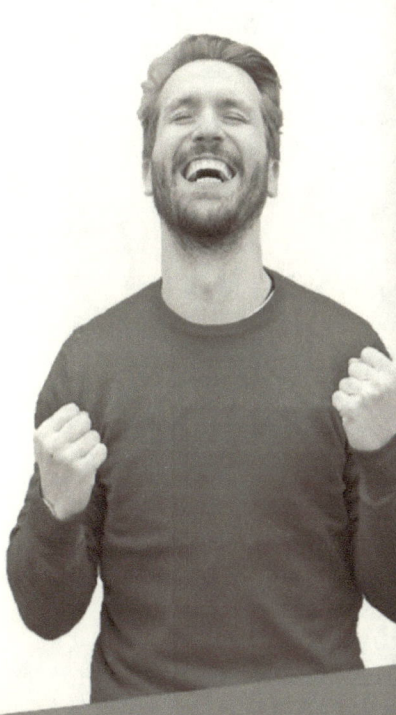

DAY 11
AFFIRMATION

Meditate on 1 Peter 2:24B in your heart for 5 minutes

"..By His stripes ye have been healed.."

Now say the words below to yourself

"I HAVE BEEN HEALED THEREFORE, I AFFIRM THAT I AM NOT DEPRESSED!"

DAY 12
AFFIRMATION

Meditate on 1 Peter 2:24B in your heart for 5 minutes

"..By His stripes ye have been healed.."

Now say the words below to yourself

"I HAVE BEEN HEALED THEREFORE, I AFFIRM THAT MY MIND IS NOT UNDER DEMONIC OPPRESSIONS!"

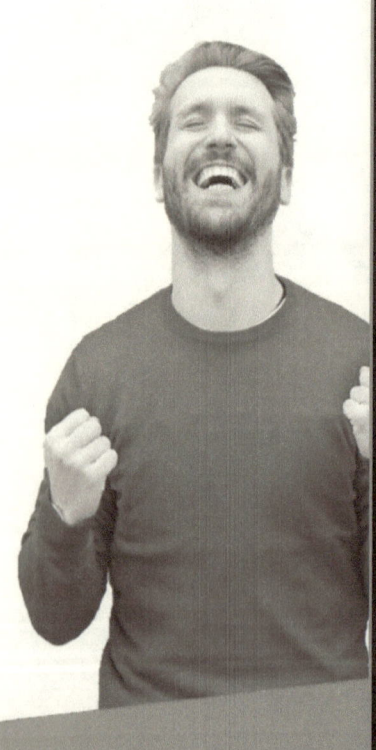

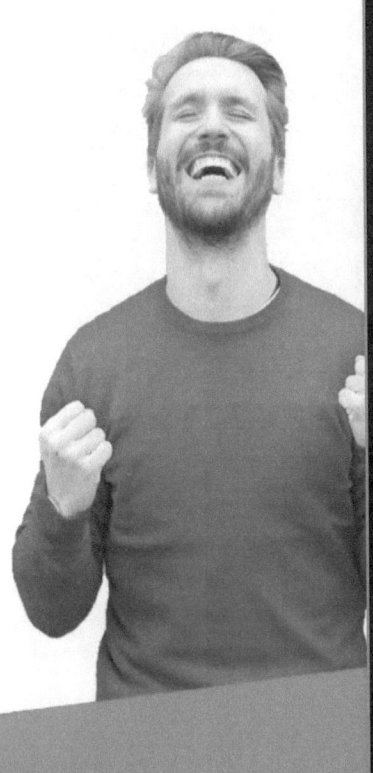

DAY 13
AFFIRMATION

Meditate on 1 Peter 2:24B in your heart for 5 minutes

"..By His stripes ye have been healed.."

Now say the words below to yourself

"I HAVE BEEN HEALED THEREFORE, I AFFIRM THAT MY LIFE IS ACTIVE AND BLESSED FOREVER!"

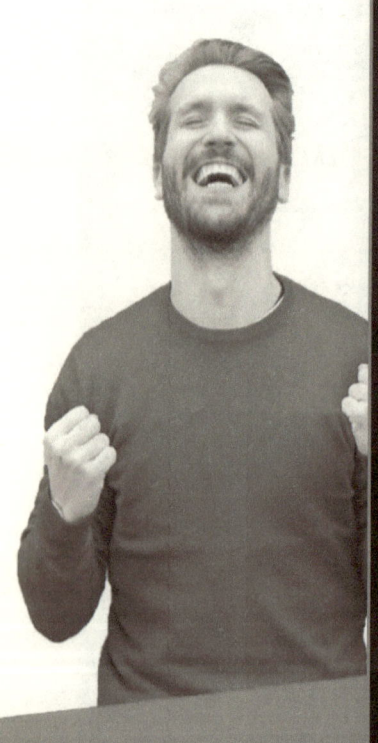

DAY 14
AFFIRMATION

Meditate on 1 Peter 2:24B in your heart for 5 minutes

"..By His stripes ye have been healed.."

Now say the words below to yourself

"I HAVE BEEN HEALED THEREFORE, I AFFIRM THAT MY FUTURE IS ACTIVE AND BLESSED FOREVER!"

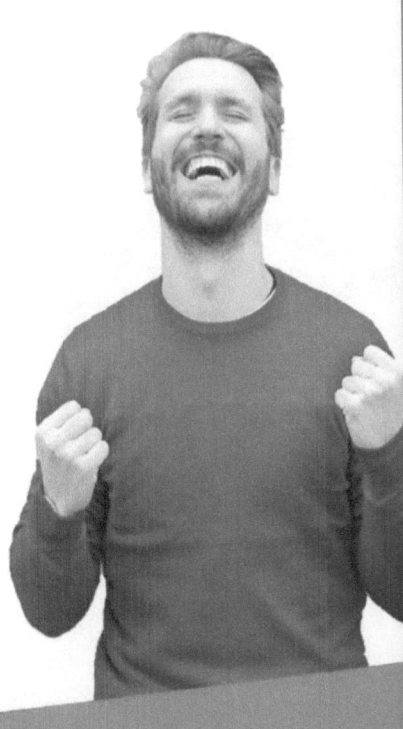

DAY 15 AFFIRMATION

Meditate on 1 Peter 2:24B in your heart for 5 minutes

"..By His stripes ye have been healed.."

Now say the words below to yourself

"I HAVE BEEN HEALED THEREFORE, I AFFIRM THAT I AM NOT DEPRESSED!"

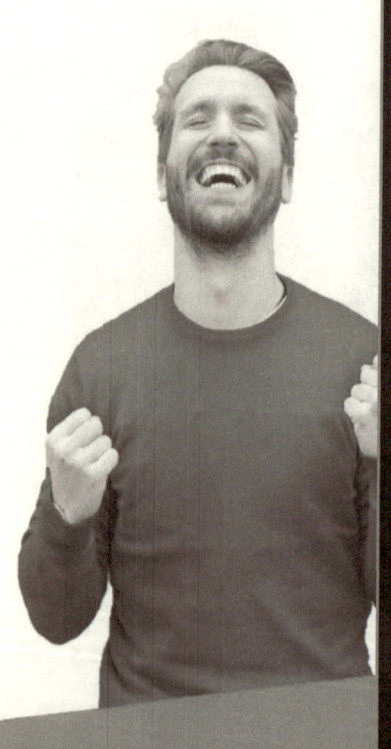

DAY 16
AFFIRMATION

Meditate on 1 Peter 2:24B in your heart for 5 minutes

"..By His stripes ye have been healed.."

Now say the words below to yourself

"I HAVE BEEN HEALED THEREFORE, I AFFIRM THAT MY MIND IS NOT UNDER SATANIC INFLUENCES!"

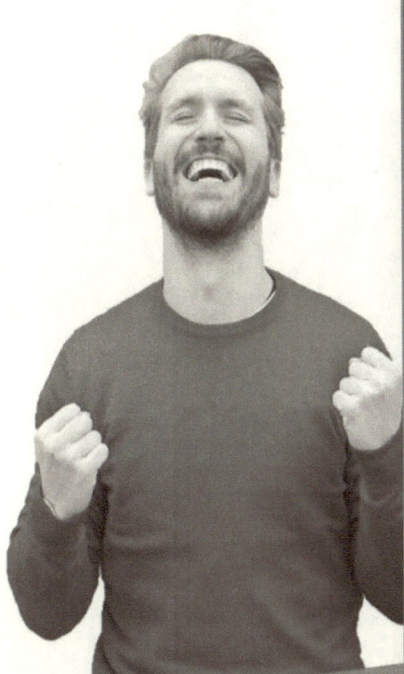

DAY 17
AFFIRMATION

Meditate on 1 Peter 2:24B in your heart for 5 minutes

"..By His stripes ye have been healed.."

Now say the words below to yourself

"I HAVE BEEN HEALED THEREFORE, I AFFIRM THAT I AM NOT DEPRESSED!"

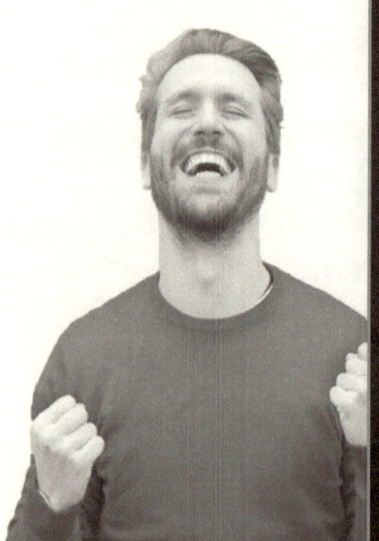

DAY 18
AFFIRMATION

Meditate on 1 Peter 2:24B in your heart for 5 minutes

"..By His stripes ye have been healed.."

Now say the words below to yourself

"MY FAMILY HAVE BEEN HEALED THEREFORE, I AFFIRM THAT MY FAMILY IS BLESSED, ACTIVE AND FRUITFUL FOREVER!"

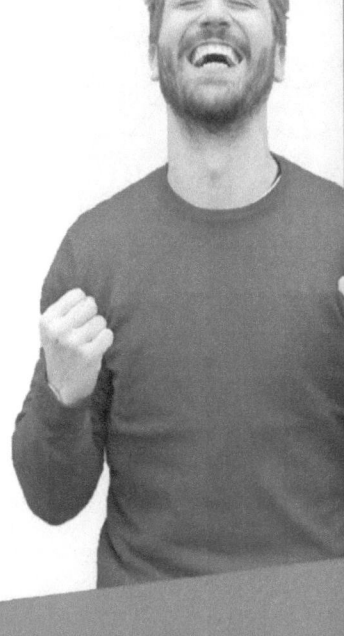

DAY 19
AFFIRMATION

Meditate on 1 Peter 2:24B in your heart for 5 minutes

"..By His stripes ye have been healed.."

Now say the words below to yourself

"I HAVE BEEN HEALED THEREFORE, I AFFIRM THAT MY FUTURE IS ACTIVE AND BLESSED FOREVER!"

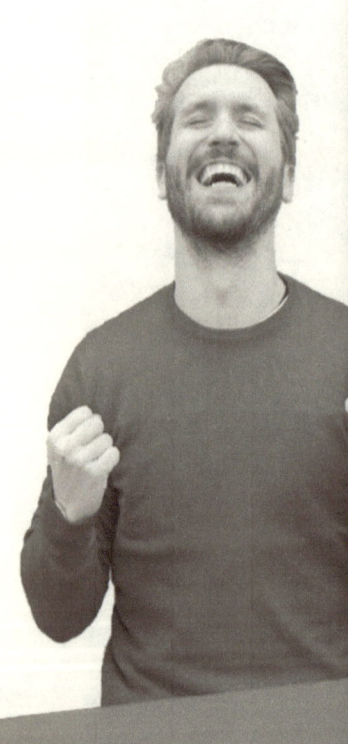

DAY 20 AFFIRMATION

Meditate on 1 Peter 2:24B in your heart for 5 minutes

"..By His stripes ye have been healed.."

Now say the words below to yourself

"I HAVE BEEN HEALED THEREFORE, I AFFIRM THAT I AM ACTIVE AND STRONG FOREVER!"

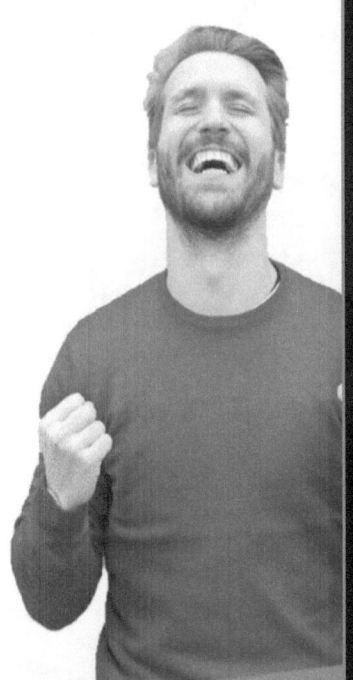

DAY 21
AFFIRMATION

Meditate on 1 Peter 2:24B in your heart for 5 minutes

"..By His stripes ye have been healed.."

Now say the words below to yourself

"I HAVE BEEN HEALED THEREFORE, I AFFIRM THAT SATAN IS A LIAR!"

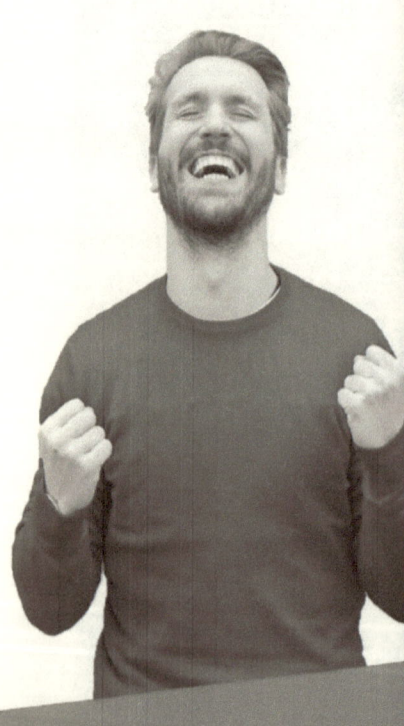

DAY 22 AFFIRMATION

Meditate on 1 Peter 2:24B in your heart for 5 minutes

"..By His stripes ye have been healed.."

Now say the words below to yourself

"I HAVE BEEN HEALED THEREFORE, I AFFIRM THAT I AM NOT DEPRESSED!"

DAY 23
AFFIRMATION

Meditate on 1 Peter 2:24B in your heart for 5 minutes

"..By His stripes ye have been healed.."

Now say the words below to yourself

"I HAVE BEEN HEALED THEREFORE, I AFFIRM THAT I AM FREE FROM ALL SATANIC MANIPULATIONS AND LIARS FOREVER!"

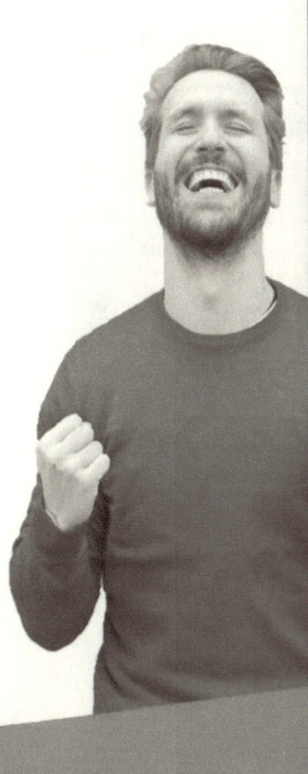

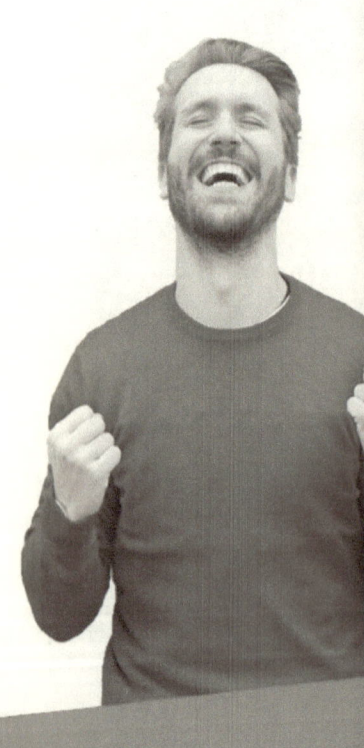

DAY 24
AFFIRMATION

Meditate on 1 Peter 2:24B in your heart for 5 minutes

"..By His stripes ye have been healed.."

Now say the words below to yourself

"I HAVE BEEN HEALED THEREFORE, I AFFIRM THAT SATAN CANNOT MAKE ME TO DESTROY MYSELF!"

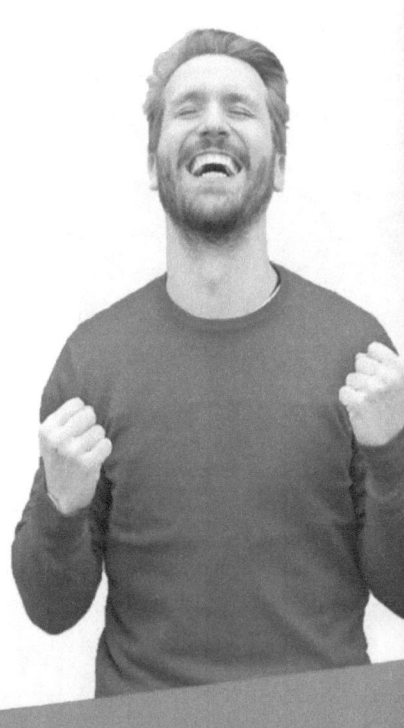

DAY 25 AFFIRMATION

Meditate on 1 Peter 2:24B in your heart for 5 minutes

"..By His stripes ye have been healed.."

Now say the words below to yourself

"I HAVE BEEN HEALED THEREFORE, I AFFIRM THAT I AM NOT DEPRESSED!"

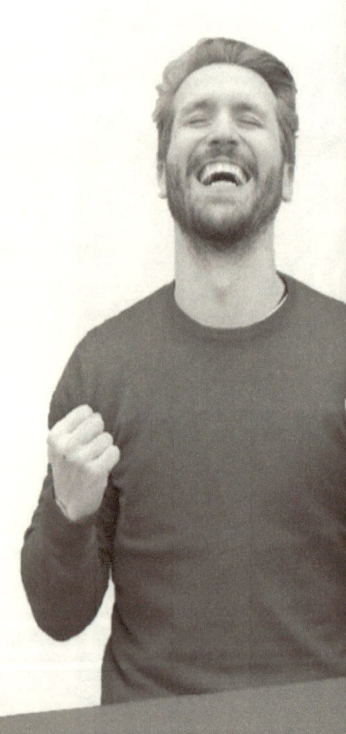

DAY 26
AFFIRMATION

Meditate on 1 Peter 2:24B in your heart for 5 minutes

"..By His stripes ye have been healed.."

Now say the words below to yourself

"I HAVE BEEN HEALED THEREFORE, I AFFIRM THAT MY LIFE IS ACTIVE AND BLESSED FOREVER!"

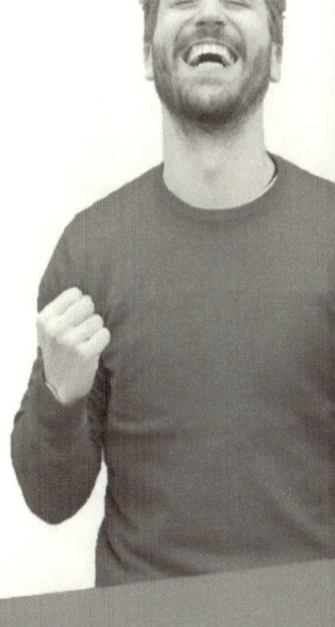

DAY 27
AFFIRMATION

Meditate on 1 Peter 2:24B in your heart for 5 minutes

"..By His stripes ye have been healed.."

Now say the words below to yourself

"I HAVE BEEN HEALED THEREFORE, I AFFIRM THAT MY BODY IS ACTIVE AND STRONG FOREVER!"

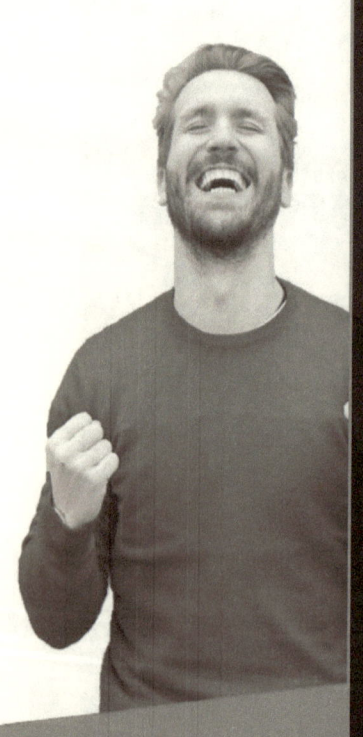

DAY 28
AFFIRMATION

Meditate on 1 Peter 2:24B in your heart for 5 minutes

"..By His stripes ye have been healed.."

Now say the words below to yourself

"I HAVE BEEN HEALED THEREFORE, I AFFIRM THAT MY FUTURE IS ACTIVE AND BLESSED FOREVER!"

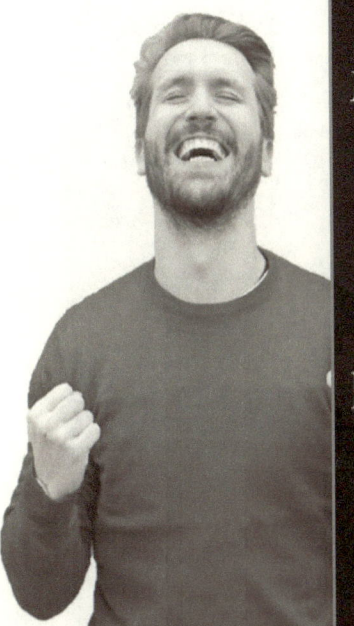

DAY 29
AFFIRMATION

Meditate on 1 Peter 2:24B in your heart for 5 minutes

"..By His stripes ye have been healed.."

Now say the words below to yourself

"I HAVE BEEN HEALED THEREFORE, I AFFIRM THAT I AM FREE FOREVER!"

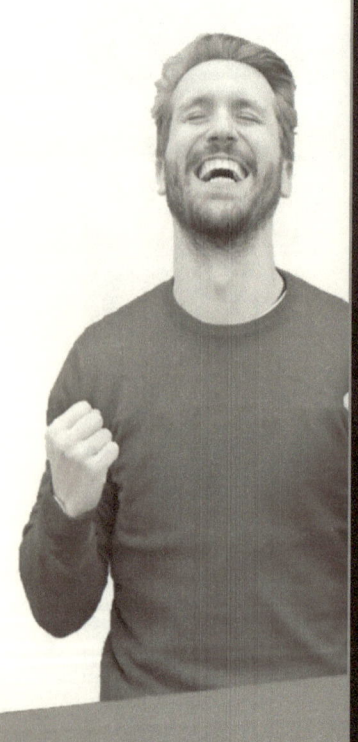

DAY 30
AFFIRMATION

Meditate on 1 Peter 2:24B in your heart for 5 minutes

"..By His stripes ye have been healed.."

Now say the words below to yourself

"MY FAMILY HAVE BEEN HEALED THEREFORE, I AFFIRM THAT MY FAMILY IS FREE FOREVER!"

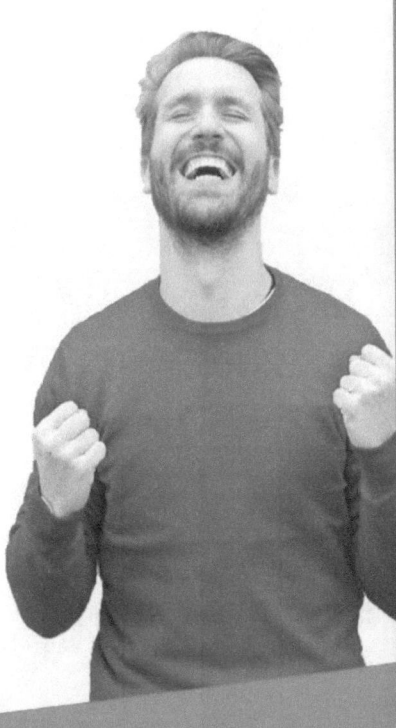

DAY 31
AFFIRMATION

Meditate on 1 Peter 2:24B in your heart for 5 minutes

"..By His stripes ye have been healed.."

Now say the following words to yourself

"I HAVE BEEN HEALED THEREFORE, I AFFIRM THAT MY LIFE AND MY FUTURE IS BLESSED, ACTIVE AND STRONG FOREVER. I AFFIRM THAT I AM NOT DEPRESSED!"

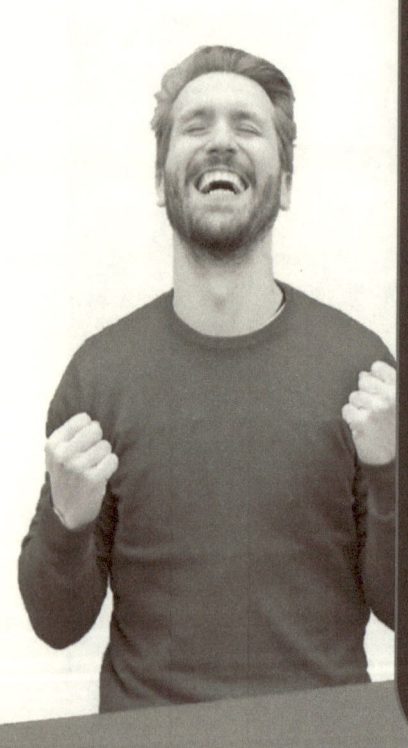

DON'T allow Satan to lie to you or deceive you.

DON'T allow demons to influence/manipulate your mind against God and against yourself.

YOU are valuable and blessed Forever because you are the child of God.

YOU have been healed and so you are free FOREVER.
(1 Peter 2:24)

LIVE IN PEACE AND JOY FOREVER!!

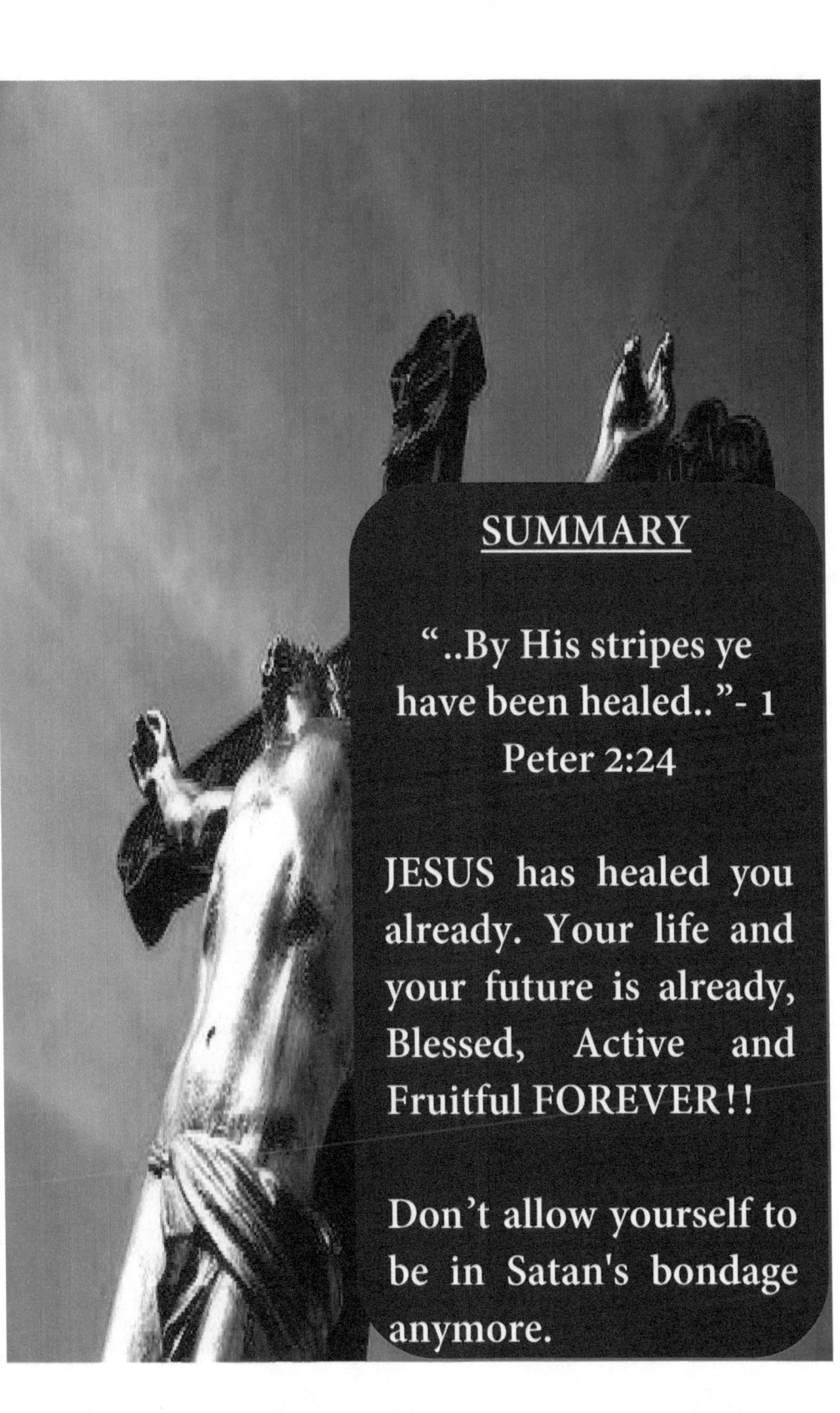

SUMMARY

"..By His stripes ye have been healed.."- 1 Peter 2:24

JESUS has healed you already. Your life and your future is already, Blessed, Active and Fruitful FOREVER!!

Don't allow yourself to be in Satan's bondage anymore.

PRAYER FOR SALVATION

We believe that you have been blessed and that you want to receive eternal life that God has made available to everyone who believes in his love and his grace which He expressed lavishly through His Son Jesus Christ.

"For God so loved the world, that He gave his only begotten Son, that whosoever <u>believeth</u> in him should not perish, but <u>have everlasting life</u>." - John 3:16

Say this prayer to God and believe it with your heart

"Father, I believe that you gave me your only Son to die for my sin. I believe you raised Him from the dead. I declare that your son, Jesus Christ is the Lord of my life. I receive eternal life and I receive the Holy Spirit. I am saved forever.in Jesus name. I am so Happy that today and forever, I am your child. Amen ".

Congratulations, you are now a child of God Halleluyah!! – John 1:12

OTHER INFORMATION

Please share your testimonies via the following handles;

ihekewilliams@gmail.com
+2348061530541

Other Books written by the author includes
Dad, Pray for your Daughter
Mum, Pray for your Daughter
Mum, pray for your Son
Don't stop the flow of the Blessing
Daddy's Prayers
Mummy's Prayers
Divine Health Affirmations Series
Divine Health Affirmations against HIV

ABOUT THE AUTHOR

Iheke Williams is a firm follower and disciple of the Lord Jesus Christ. He is a passionate minister of the grace of our Lord and savior Jesus Christ and has brought the reality of the divine life of Christ into the lives of so many.

Iheke Williams has a calling to communicate the gospel of Christ with simplicity and to show the world how to activate the eternal life of God that is in us already which includes Divine health, Divine righteousness, Divine security and Divine prosperity.

As you read this book and other books written by Iheke Williams you will literally begin to function and manifest the life of God that is already inside you to the glory of God the Father who is the author of all grace and mercy. Amen!

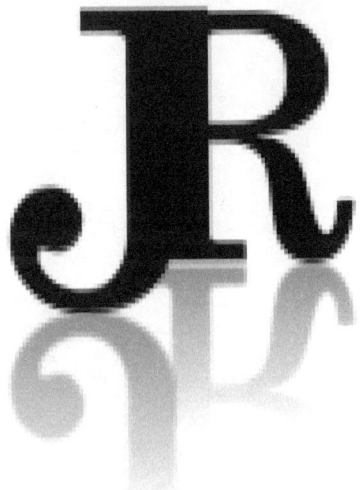

www.ingramcontent.com/pod-product-compliance
Lightning Source LLC
Chambersburg PA
CBHW021939170526
45157CB00005B/2353